# KNOWLEDGE GUIDE TO
# RHEUMATOID
# ARTHRITIS

Essential Manual To Proven Strategies, Pain Relief, And Effective Treatments For Joint Health

DR. AARON BRANUM

Copyright © 2024 BY DR. AARON BRANUM

All rights reserved. Except for brief quotations embodied in critical reviews and certain other noncommercial uses permitted by copyright law, no part of this publication may be reproduced, distributed, or transmitted in any form or by any means, Including photocopying, recording, or other electronic or mechanical methods, without the prior written permission of the publisher.

## Disclaimer:

The data in this book, is solely meant to be informative and instructional.

This book is not intended to replace expert medical advice, diagnosis, or care. No medical, health, or other professional services are offered by the author, publisher, or any affiliated parties

Individual outcomes may differ in the practice of these therapies, which entail a variety of approaches and methodologies.

A one-on-one session with a trained or certified healthcare professional is still preferable. It is best to consult a trained healthcare provider before making any decisions regarding your health.

The author of this book is not affiliated with any specific website, product, or organization related to any of these therapies.

All reasonable measures have been taken by the author and publisher to guarantee the authenticity and dependability of the material contained in this book

**Contents**

**CHAPTER ONE**..............................................15

  **DIAGNOSIS AND SYMPTOMS** ....................15

    Identifying Rheumatoid Arthritis Symptoms: ...................................................................15

    Recognizing The Role Of Medical Professionals In Diagnosis: .....................16

    The Value Of An Early And Precise Diagnosis ...................................................................17

**CHAPTER TWO** ............................................19

  **OPTIONS FOR TREATMENT** .......................19

    Drugs For Treating The Symptoms Of Rheumatoid Arthritis: ...........................19

    Modifications To Lifestyle And Self-Care Techniques: ............................................20

    Occupational And Physical Therapy: ........21

    Surgical Procedures For More Serious Situations: ..........................................22

    Alternative And Complementary Therapies: ...................................................................23

**CHAPTER THREE** ........................................25

  **MANAGEMENT OF DISEASES** ...................25

Formulating A Successful Treatment Strategy ................................................25

Pain And Fatigue Coping Mechanisms.......27

The Value Of A Healthy Lifestyle And Frequent Exercise ..................................29

Support For Mental Health......................32

## CHAPTER FOUR .........................................35

### COPING WITH ARTHRITIS RHEUMATOID ....35

Strategies For Handling Everyday Tasks With Rheumatoid Arthritis ......................35

Establishing A Cosy And Accessible Living Space.................................................37

Techniques For Preserving Self-Sufficiency And Mobility .........................................38

Handling Communication And Relationship Issues ................................................40

Resources And Rheumatoid Arthritis Support Systems For Individuals ........................41

## CHAPTER FIVE ..........................................45

### RHEUMATOID ARTHRITIS AND NUTRITION .45

Recognizing The Function Of Diet ............45

Foods To Take And Leave Out.................45

    Maintaining a Healthy Weight Is Crucial ...46

    Supplemental Nutrition And Its Possible Advantages ............................................. 47

    Speaking With A Certified Dietitian .......... 48

CHAPTER SIX .................................................. 49

  GYNAECOLOGY AND ARTHRITIS OF THE PUMP ........................................................................ 49

    Handling The Symptoms Of Rheumatoid Arthritis During Pregnancy ..................... 49

    Pregnancy-Related Risks And Things To Think About When Taking Medication ....... 52

    Prenatal Care And Preconception Planning Are Important ........................................ 56

    Coping Strategies For Expectant Patients With Rheumatoid Arthritis ...................... 59

    Rheumatoid Arthritis And Breastfeeding: Postpartum Considerations ..................... 62

CHAPTER SEVEN ............................................. 67

  RHEUMATOID ARTHRITIS AND WORK ........ 67

    Workplace Rights And Accommodations ... 67

    Techniques For Handling Stress And Fatigue Associated With Work ........................... 68

Interacting With Coworkers And Employers .................................................. 69
Benefits For Disability And Flexible Work Schedules .............................................. 70
Juggling Work-Related Obligations With Treatment And Self-Care........................ 71

# CHAPTER EIGHT ........................................ 73
## SCIENCE AND FUTURE POSSIBILITIES ....... 73
Current Research On Rheumatoid Arthritis Trends And Developments...................... 73
Potential Treatment Strategies In The Works .................................................................. 75
Clinical Trials' Significance In Promoting Rheumatoid Arthritis Treatment .............. 76
Campaigning And Collecting Money For Rheumatoid Arthritis Research ................ 78
Prospects For Enhanced Results And Life Quality For Patients With Rheumatoid Arthritis In The Future .......................... 79

# CHAPTER NINE............................................ 83
## COMMONLY ASKED QUESTIONS OR FAQS .. 83
How Does Rheumatoid Arthritis Develop? . 83

Does Rheumatoid Arthritis Run In Families? ...................................................... 85

Is There A Cure For Rheumatoid Arthritis? 86

How Should I Handle Flare-Ups Of My Rheumatoid Arthritis? ............................ 88

If I Think I May Have Rheumatoid Arthritis, What Should I Do? ........................... 90

## ABOUT THIS BOOK

The "Knowledge Guide to Rheumatoid Arthritis" is an invaluable resource for anyone attempting to make sense of the complicated world of this autoimmune disease. Its foundation is an educational introduction, which is essential to understanding the complexities of Rheumatoid Arthritis (RA). It explores the central query: what precisely is RA? It dispels myths that frequently skew perception and lays out the main differences between RA and other types of arthritis, laying the groundwork for a more thorough investigation.

The chapters on symptoms and diagnosis are crucial because they provide a path toward awareness and comprehension. This section provides readers with the skills to actively engage with healthcare providers in pursuit of an accurate diagnosis—a crucial first step towards optimal management—from recognizing subtle indications to navigating diagnostic procedures.

A range of options are available for treatment, ranging from pharmacological interventions to comprehensive lifestyle modifications. Along with insights into the possibilities of surgical procedures and the function of complementary therapies, readers are guided through the terrain of pharmaceutical management. Based on the principles of patient-centered care, this section emphasizes the value of team decision-making when creating customized treatment programs.

The pivotal role of Disease Management is highlighted, stressing the dynamic interaction between attentive observation and flexible tactics. People can handle the ups and downs of RA with grace and resilience by integrating mental health support and using effective coping methods.

The focus is on living with rheumatoid arthritis, which provides a road plan for regaining independence and energy in spite of obstacles. This section acts as a guide for creating a life full of possibilities and significance, from streamlining daily tasks to cultivating deep connections.

Nutrition and Rheumatoid Arthritis shed light on the significant influence that dietary decisions have on managing symptoms and highlighting the importance of nutrition as a foundational element of overall well-being. By providing readers with useful advice on dietary adjustments and the incorporation of nutritional supplements, they may fully utilize food's healing potential.

Pregnancy and Rheumatoid Arthritis deftly negotiate the confluence of chronic illness and parenting, providing valuable perspectives on the particular factors and networks of support that are critical to the health of mothers.

For those juggling the demands of their jobs and their health, the combination of work with rheumatoid arthritis provides a lifeline. This part supports the right to meaningful and happy employment by promoting workplace adjustments and finding a healthy balance between career goals and self-care.

Research and Future Directions traces the path of invention and discovery in the field of RA with an optimistic eye toward the future. Readers are encouraged to join the movement for better results and a higher standard of living by viewing it through the lenses of advocacy and community involvement.

Frequently Asked Questions (FAQs) provide a clear reference point by skillfully and sympathetically answering frequently asked questions. This section demystifies the challenges of living with RA, promoting empowerment through knowledge and solving some of the mysteries surrounding the disease's beginnings as well as providing useful tactics for managing flares.

# CHAPTER ONE

## DIAGNOSIS AND SYMPTOMS

### Identifying Rheumatoid Arthritis Symptoms:

Rheumatoid arthritis usually affects smaller joints first, such as the hands and feet, and frequently presents as joint pain, stiffness, and swelling.

There may be fluctuations in the onset, severity, and length of symptoms. It is imperative that chronic pain be taken seriously, particularly in the morning or following periods of inactivity.

Diagnostic Tests and Procedures: A physical examination, a medical history, and specialized tests are used to diagnose rheumatoid arthritis. Anti-cyclic citrullinated peptide (anti-CCP) antibodies and rheumatoid factor (RF) blood tests aid in the confirmation of the diagnosis. Joint inflammation and injury are also evaluated using imaging procedures like X-rays and ultrasounds.

## Recognizing The Role Of Medical Professionals In Diagnosis:

Rheumatologists, general practitioners, and nurses are among the medical professionals who are essential in the diagnosis of Rheumatoid Arthritis. Specialized in autoimmune diseases such as RA, rheumatologists play a crucial role in the interpretation of test data, formulation of therapy recommendations, and tracking the course of the disease.

Making the Distinction Between Rheumatoid Arthritis and Other Conditions:

Accurate diagnosis of rheumatoid arthritis is difficult since it shares symptoms with other forms of arthritis and autoimmune illnesses. However certain traits, such as symmetrical joint involvement, and rheumatoid nodules, can help differentiate RA from other illnesses like lupus or osteoarthritis.

## The Value Of An Early And Precise Diagnosis

Effective care and joint damage prevention of Rheumatoid Arthritis depend on an early and precise diagnosis. Early intervention with lifestyle modifications and disease-modifying drugs can help reduce disability and joint deformities, regulate symptoms, and enhance quality of life.

# CHAPTER TWO

## OPTIONS FOR TREATMENT

### Drugs For Treating The Symptoms Of Rheumatoid Arthritis:

Rheumatoid arthritis (RA) is treated with a variety of drugs. Ibuprofen is one example of a nonsteroidal anti-inflammatory medicine (NSAID) that can help lessen pain and inflammation. In order to maintain joint function and slow down the progression of RA, doctors frequently administer disease-modifying antirheumatic medications (DMARDs), such as methotrexate.

To lessen inflammation and joint injury, biological medicines, such as TNF-alpha inhibitors, target particular immune system components. During flare-ups, corticosteroids may also be administered to treat symptoms fast.

## Modifications To Lifestyle And Self-Care Techniques:

To effectively manage rheumatoid arthritis, lifestyle modifications, and self-care techniques are essential in addition to medication. Frequent exercise helps enhance muscle strength, joint flexibility, and general fitness. Low-impact exercises like cycling or swimming can help with this.

Retaining a healthy weight can help alleviate pain and inflammation by easing the strain on joints. Sufficient sleep coupled with stress-reduction methods like deep breathing exercises or meditation can help reduce symptoms and improve general health.

Additionally, reducing alcohol intake and giving up smoking can help with RA symptoms.

## Occupational And Physical Therapy:

Essential to managing RA is physical and occupational therapy, which aims to enhance joint function, mobility, and overall quality of life.

To increase joint range of motion, strengthen muscles, and promote flexibility, physical therapists create customized workout regimens. Occupational therapists offer methods and assistive technology to lessen the strain on afflicted joints and simplify daily duties. The goal of these therapies is to enable people with RA to continue being independent and partake in worthwhile activities in spite of their illness.

## Surgical Procedures For More Serious Situations:

Surgical operations may be required in severe cases of rheumatoid arthritis when conservative therapy is insufficient to relieve the condition's symptoms.

In severely injured joints, joint replacement surgery (e.g., hip or knee replacement) can relieve discomfort and restore mobility.

To lessen inflammation and delay the degeneration of the joints, a synovectomy—the removal of the inflammatory synovial tissue lining the joints—may be carried out.

For those with advanced RA, surgical interventions are intended to increase overall quality of life, reduce discomfort, and improve joint function.

## Alternative And Complementary Therapies:

Many people with rheumatoid arthritis look into complementary and alternative therapies in addition to traditional treatments in order to better control their symptoms. These could consist of nutritional adjustments, herbal supplements, massage therapy, and acupuncture. Although there is little scientific proof that these treatments are helpful for treating RA, some people find them to be helpful for managing their symptoms and generally feeling better. It's crucial to talk to a healthcare professional about any complementary or alternative therapies to make sure they work in tandem with traditional RA treatments rather than against them.

# CHAPTER THREE

## MANAGEMENT OF DISEASES

### Formulating A Successful Treatment Strategy

Creating a thorough treatment plan with your medical team is one of the most important things you can do to manage your rheumatoid arthritis (RA). Typically, this strategy consists of a mix of prescription drugs, dietary adjustments, and specially designed therapies. To decide on the best course of action, your healthcare professional will evaluate a number of criteria, including the intensity of your symptoms, your general health, and any pre-existing medical issues.

The mainstay of treatment for RA is frequent medication. Prescriptions for biologic agents, DMARDs, and nonsteroidal anti-inflammatory medications (NSAIDs) are frequently written in an effort to relieve pain, lower inflammation, and slow the course of illness. Corticosteroids are another medication that your doctor could use to give temporary relief during flare-ups.

Adjusting one's lifestyle is essential to controlling RA in addition to medicine. This could entail avoiding activities that worsen symptoms, keeping a healthy weight to lessen stress on your joints, and implementing a balanced diet full of foods that are anti-inflammatory. Enhancing joint function and mobility might also benefit from physical and occupational therapy.

To make sure that your treatment strategy continues to work, it is imperative that you regularly examine the course of the condition. It's likely that your doctor may arrange for

...aller, more manageable segments. You can ...so lessen the pressure on your body and save ...ergy by learning to assign duties to others ...d seek for assistance when necessary.

...art from managing your schedule, employing ...ethods of relaxation like deep breathing, ...editation, or guided imagery can aid in ...ducing tension and fostering calmness. These ...thods can be especially helpful when you're ...ling more tired or in pain.

...en done properly, physical activity can also ... in reducing RA-related discomfort and ...gue. Exercises that don't put too much ...in on your joints, like swimming, cycling, or ...a, can build your muscles, develop ...urance, and improve joint flexibility. You ... create an exercise program that is safe and ...ient and customized to your unique

routine examinations and testing in
evaluate your condition and mo
treatment plan as needed. Any chan
general health or symptoms
discussed honestly with your docto
help them make necessary modi
your treatment plan.

## Pain And Fatigue Coping Mec

RA can be difficult to live with, esp
it comes to wearing off and ma
Thankfully, you may enhance
quality of life and effectively m
symptoms with the use of a num
mechanisms.

Above all, it's critical to pace yo
attention to your body. This
prioritizing chores according to
taking regular pauses, and divi

requirements and abilities by working with a physical therapist or professional fitness instructor.

Lastly, when coping with the difficulties of RA, asking for help from friends, family, or a support group can offer both practical and emotional support. It can be tremendously encouraging to share experiences and coping mechanisms with people who are familiar with your situation and to feel less alone while navigating the disease.

## The Value Of A Healthy Lifestyle And Frequent Exercise

Keeping up a consistent exercise schedule and living a healthy lifestyle is crucial for both controlling rheumatoid arthritis (RA) and enhancing general well-being. Frequent exercise can help strengthen and increase flexibility while also reducing stiffness and soreness in the joints.

It's crucial to select joint-friendly exercises for your fitness regimen that won't make your symptoms worse. People with RA can usually manage low-impact exercises like yoga, walking, cycling, and swimming. Without putting undue strain on your joints, these exercises assist in strengthening your muscles, enhance your cardiovascular health, and boost your general mobility.

Adopting a healthy lifestyle can enhance your general health and well-being even more than exercising. In addition to providing vital nutrients to promote joint health, a balanced diet full of fruits, vegetables, whole grains, and lean proteins can help reduce inflammation. Reducing inflammation and enhancing general health can also be achieved by avoiding processed foods, high sugar, and bad fats.

For those who have RA, maintaining a healthy weight is especially crucial because being overweight can worsen symptoms by putting undue strain on the joints. Even a tiny weight loss can have a big impact on joint discomfort and function if you're fat or overweight.

A healthy lifestyle also includes stress management and obtaining enough sleep, in addition to exercise and a balanced diet. Discovering appropriate coping mechanisms for chronic stress, such as mindfulness practices, relaxation techniques, or enjoyable hobbies, can assist enhance your general well-being because chronic stress can worsen inflammation and pain. In a similar vein, making sleep a priority and maintaining appropriate sleep hygiene helps lessen fatigue and increase your capacity to manage the difficulties associated with RA.

## Support For Mental Health

Living with rheumatoid arthritis (RA) can be mentally taxing due to the condition's weariness, physical restrictions, and chronic pain, which can be difficult to deal with emotionally. You can enhance your overall quality of life and more effectively manage the emotional effects of RA by seeking mental health support and learning coping mechanisms.

Developing an optimistic outlook and engaging in self-compassion exercises are crucial coping mechanisms. Changing your perspective and enhancing your general view of life can be accomplished by learning to accept your limitations, concentrate on the things within your control, and enjoy incremental successes. Creating attainable objectives and working towards them can also boost self-esteem and emotions of achievement.

Seeking assistance from friends, family, or a mental health professional can offer helpful emotional support and encouragement in addition to self-care techniques. Open communication about your emotions and experiences with people you can trust can reduce feelings of loneliness and foster understanding and a sense of connection.

Joining online forums or support groups for RA sufferers can also be helpful because they give a secure setting for exchanging helpful advice, experiences, and encouragement with one another. Making connections with people who are cognizant of your experiences can alleviate feelings of isolation and offer support and affirmation.

Don't be afraid to get professional assistance from a therapist or counselor who specializes in chronic disease or pain management if you're finding it difficult to handle the emotional effects of RA.

Therapy can help you handle the difficulties of having RA and enhance your quality of life overall by teaching you coping mechanisms, stress-reduction methods, and emotional support.

# CHAPTER FOUR

## COPING WITH ARTHRITIS RHEUMATOID

### Strategies For Handling Everyday Tasks With Rheumatoid Arthritis

Although rheumatoid arthritis (RA) can make daily tasks difficult, there are techniques to assist you in efficiently managing your activities. First and foremost, it's critical to set priorities for your work and divide it into smaller, more doable pieces. By doing this, you may avoid overdoing it and maintain your energy levels throughout the day. Pacing oneself is also essential. Take breaks when necessary and pay attention to your body to avoid overstretching yourself.

It's crucial to modify your everyday activities to take your condition into account. Consider employing assistive gadgets or products that can make activities easier, such as ergonomic utensils for cooking or jar openers for opening resistant lids.

Another important change you can make is to arrange your home to put as little stress on your joints as possible. Invest in comfortable, accessible furnishings and equipment, and keep commonly used goods easily accessible.

Additionally, using proper body mechanics and posture will assist reduce joint stress and stop additional suffering. Try to distribute your weight evenly and move with awareness to prevent overstressing any one joint. You can also lessen stiffness and increase flexibility by adding mild stretching and strengthening exercises to your everyday regimen.

## Establishing A Cosy And Accessible Living Space

Creating a comfortable and easily accessible living space is crucial for the management of rheumatoid arthritis. Make sure everything in your house is clear of clutter and anything that can cause you to trip or fall. To give further support and stability, think about putting grab bars and handrails in places like the lavatory and stairwell.

Purchasing ergonomic items and furniture will help improve your comfort and lessen joint stress. Select couches and chairs that will support your arms and back well, and use pillows or cushions to offer more cushioning where it's needed. Additionally, you can adapt your surroundings to meet your unique demands by utilizing accessories and furniture with adjustable heights.

Throughout your house, create specific spaces for relaxation to help you save energy and prevent overdoing. Provide cozy places to sit and decompress, and think about adding features like calming music and soft lighting to encourage relaxation. Simple adjustments like installing tap controls and door handles with levers can help simplify and manage everyday chores.

## Techniques For Preserving Self-Sufficiency And Mobility

Sustaining autonomy and movement is crucial for people with rheumatoid arthritis. To do this, you must learn coping mechanisms and adaptable tactics that will provide you the confidence to face obstacles in your daily life. Prioritizing tasks according to their energy requirements and significance can be a useful tactic. This involves concentrating on the most important tasks first and assigning or delaying the less important ones as needed.

When navigating your surroundings, using mobility aids like wheelchairs, walkers, or canes can offer extra stability and support. Make sure the aids you select are suitable for your unique requirements and talents, and don't be afraid to ask occupational therapists or medical specialists for advice if you're not sure which options are ideal for you.

Regular physical exercise can also aid with rheumatoid arthritis pain and stiffness reduction, as well as mobility improvement. Select low-impact workouts like tai chi, cycling, or swimming to increase your strength and flexibility without putting too much strain on your joints. Furthermore, using proper body mechanics and posture can help lower the chance of injury and increase mobility in general.

## Handling Communication And Relationship Issues

Relationships and communication with people may be negatively impacted by having rheumatoid arthritis, but there are ways to deal with these difficulties. Being upfront and truthful with your loved ones about your illness and how it affects you is crucial because it can promote empathy and understanding. Promote open communication and don't hesitate to seek assistance when you need it.

You can preserve deep relationships with others by learning how to cope with pain and exhaustion during social situations. Keep a healthy pace, provide your top priorities, and don't be afraid to establish boundaries or take breaks when necessary. In addition, think about asking friends and family for assistance with chores and activities that might be too much for you to handle alone.

Finding rheumatoid arthritis support groups or online communities can be a great way to get both practical guidance for overcoming the condition's obstacles and emotional support. Making connections with people who are aware of your experiences helps lessen feelings of loneliness and foster a sense of community and friendship.

## Resources And Rheumatoid Arthritis Support Systems For Individuals

Managing rheumatoid arthritis and overcoming its obstacles can be made easier by finding resources and support systems. Make initial contact with medical specialists who treat RA, such as rheumatologists, physical therapists, and occupational therapists. They can offer helpful advice and assistance that is catered to your unique requirements and situation.

In addition, rheumatoid arthritis sufferers and their families can get assistance from a plethora of advocacy groups and organizations. These groups frequently provide community gatherings, support groups, and educational materials with the goal of educating the public and building relationships among individuals impacted by the illness.

Use these tools to connect with others who can provide compassion and empathy and to learn more about managing RA.

For those with rheumatoid arthritis, online tools including reliable websites, forums, and social media groups can also offer helpful information and support. Be cautious to look for trustworthy information sources and interact with groups that value empowerment, encouragement, and positivity.

You can get insightful information, useful advice, and emotional support to help you through the challenges of living with rheumatoid arthritis by utilizing these resources and support systems.

# CHAPTER FIVE

## RHEUMATOID ARTHRITIS AND NUTRITION

### Recognizing The Function Of Diet

In order to control the symptoms of rheumatoid arthritis (RA), diet is essential. Although there isn't a single diet that can treat RA, some foods can assist manage symptoms and enhance general health. In order to effectively manage this illness with nutrition, it is important to understand how certain nutrients affect inflammation and immunological function.

### Foods To Take And Leave Out

You can lessen inflammation and your RA symptoms by eating a diet rich in anti-inflammatory foods. These include veggies like broccoli, kale, and spinach as well as fruits like oranges, berries, and cherries. Flaxseeds, walnuts, salmon, and sardines are good sources of omega-3 fatty acids, which can also help lower inflammation.

However, it's crucial to minimize items that can aggravate RA symptoms by causing inflammation. These include processed foods that are heavy in harmful fats and refined sugars, as well as those that are high in trans and saturated fats. Cutting back on processed and red meat consumption can also be advantageous.

## Maintaining a Healthy Weight Is Crucial

For those who have rheumatoid arthritis, it's imperative to maintain a healthy weight. Being overweight strains the joints more, which exacerbates discomfort and inflammation. A balanced diet low in calorie-dense foods and high in nutrients can help people reach and maintain a healthy weight, which eases the strain on their joints.

## Supplemental Nutrition And Its Possible Advantages

For those with RA, there are certain nutritional supplements that can enhance a balanced diet and offer extra advantages. Omega-3 fatty acid supplementation, for instance, has been demonstrated to enhance joint function and lower inflammation. In a similar vein, vitamin D supplements can promote bone health, which is critical for RA patients because they may be more susceptible to osteoporosis.

Before beginning any new supplements, it's crucial to speak with a doctor because some may interfere with prescription drugs or cause other health issues.

## Speaking With A Certified Dietitian

It is strongly advised to speak with a trained dietitian for individualized nutritional guidance catered to each person's requirements and preferences. A dietitian can assist in developing a meal plan that takes into consideration any dietary restrictions and dietary sensitivities while meeting certain nutritional needs. They can also offer advice on how to maintain a long-term healthy diet, including portion amounts and scheduling of meals.

Rheumatoid arthritis sufferers can enhance their nutrition to better control their symptoms and enhance their general quality of life by consulting with a nutritionist.

# CHAPTER SIX

## GYNAECOLOGY AND ARTHRITIS OF THE PUMP

### Handling The Symptoms Of Rheumatoid Arthritis During Pregnancy

Emotions and physical changes abound during pregnancy, particularly for those with rheumatoid arthritis (RA). Even though it's a happy time, RA symptoms may be impacted by immune system changes and hormone fluctuations. However, many people can get through pregnancy with little to no health interruption if they manage their pregnancy well.

Working with your healthcare team to manage your RA throughout pregnancy is essential. This applies to your obstetrician, rheumatologist, and any other medical professionals who are treating you. They may offer advice based on your particular circumstances and guarantee that your treatment plan is secure for you and your child.

It's critical to regularly check RA symptoms throughout pregnancy. Hormonal changes during pregnancy may cause some people's symptoms to lessen, while they may worsen for others. Monitoring any changes enables timely treatment modifications when necessary.

It's crucial to keep up a healthy lifestyle when managing RA throughout pregnancy. This entails maintaining a healthy weight, controlling stress, getting enough sleep, and engaging in regular exercise as advised by your doctor. These routines may aid in better managing the symptoms of RA and promote general well-being.

Finding a balance between treating your RA symptoms and making sure your unborn child is safe throughout pregnancy is crucial.

This could entail finding safer alternatives to current medicines or modifying prescriptions. Your medical team can assist you in making these decisions by helping you balance the advantages and disadvantages of different options.

Apart from medical supervision, enlisting in support groups and asking family and friends for assistance can be quite helpful in providing emotional support for pregnant RA patients. Making connections with people who get what you're going through can reduce feelings of loneliness and offer helpful advice on how to manage RA while pregnant.

You can successfully manage RA symptoms throughout pregnancy and concentrate on the happy experience of welcoming a new member of your family by collaborating closely with your healthcare team, leading a healthy lifestyle, and asking for help when needed.

## Pregnancy-Related Risks And Things To Think About When Taking Medication

Medication management for rheumatoid arthritis (RA) patients who are pregnant or intend to become pregnant needs to be carefully considered.

Although managing the symptoms of RA is crucial for the health and welfare of mothers, the safety of pharmaceuticals during pregnancy is the main issue.

One of the difficulties is that a lot of the conventional RA drugs, such as leflunomide and methotrexate, are not advised to be taken while pregnant since they may affect the growing fetus.

In order to appropriately control RA symptoms during pregnancy, these drugs are frequently stopped before conception and substitute therapy is investigated.

Due to possible hazards to the developing baby's heart and kidneys, nonsteroidal anti-inflammatory medicines (NSAIDs), which are frequently used to treat RA symptoms, are typically not advised during the third trimester.

Under the supervision of a healthcare professional, several NSAIDs may be used cautiously during the first and second trimesters, though.

Prednisone is one of the corticosteroids that are frequently used to treat RA flare-ups during pregnancy because, when taken at low doses for brief periods of time, they can quickly relieve symptoms with little risk to the fetus.

On the other hand, prolonged usage of corticosteroids during pregnancy can increase the risk of low birth weight and premature delivery.

TNF inhibitors and other targeted therapies are examples of biological drugs that are being used more often to treat RA and are thought to be quite safe for some women to take while pregnant.

The decision to continue or stop taking biologics during pregnancy should be determined case-by-case after considering the advantages and disadvantages, given there is a lack of information regarding the long-term effects of these drugs on fetal development.

Pregnant or intending-to-be RA patients should collaborate closely with their medical team to create a pharmaceutical regimen that strikes a compromise between the baby's safety and the need to control RA symptoms.

This could entail changing prescription dosages, looking into different therapies, and keeping a close eye out for any possible issues during the course of the pregnancy.

People with RA can make empowered decisions regarding the use of medications during pregnancy that prioritize the health of both the mother and the fetus by remaining informed and cooperating with healthcare practitioners.

the fetus once pregnancy is established. This entails ongoing collaboration with a rheumatologist to manage RA symptoms and drugs during pregnancy, as well as routine check-ups with an obstetrician who has experience handling high-risk pregnancies.

Extra screening and monitoring throughout pregnancy may be necessary to spot any possible issues early and take appropriate action. This could entail keeping an eye out for symptoms of gestational diabetes, preeclampsia, and other pregnancy-related issues that might be more prevalent in RA patients.

Safe pregnancy and birth are more likely for those with RA if they prioritize preconception planning and obtain thorough prenatal care. A healthy baby can be welcomed into the world and many people with RA can successfully navigate pregnancy with the help of healthcare specialists and cautious management.

## Coping Strategies For Expectant Patients With Rheumatoid Arthritis

For those who have rheumatoid arthritis (RA), pregnancy can present special challenges; nevertheless, with the correct tools and assistance, RA symptoms can be properly managed, and a healthy pregnancy can be achieved. In order to help pregnant people with RA handle this journey with confidence and peace of mind, supportive measures are essential.

Having access to a comprehensive healthcare team with expertise in managing RA and high-risk pregnancies is a crucial source of assistance. A rheumatologist, an obstetrician, a perinatologist, and other doctors who can offer complete care customized to the patient's needs may be on this team.

For pregnant RA patients, education and knowledge are also vital sources of support. This includes knowing which drugs are safe to take while pregnant, how pregnancy may influence RA symptoms, and how to successfully treat flare-ups while reducing risks to the unborn child.

Peer networks and support groups can offer helpful coping mechanisms and emotional support for managing RA during pregnancy. Developing relationships with people who are experiencing comparable things helps lessen feelings of loneliness and foster a sense of understanding and community.

Pregnant RA patients may also benefit from practical support, such as help with household chores and child care, particularly during periods when symptoms may be more difficult to control. A solid support network helps ensure that a person can concentrate on their health and well-being throughout pregnancy by reducing stress.

Self-care routines are essential for controlling RA symptoms during pregnancy, in addition to outside assistance. This entails obtaining adequate sleep, maintaining a healthy diet, engaging in physical activity within the bounds prescribed by medical professionals, and using mindfulness and relaxation techniques to reduce stress.

RA during pregnancy can be effectively managed by pregnant individuals by prioritizing self-care, getting support from peers and loved ones, and gaining access to comprehensive treatment. This allows the individual to concentrate on enjoying this unique time in their lives. It is possible to have a safe pregnancy and confidently and optimistically welcome a new member of the family with the correct support system in place.

## Rheumatoid Arthritis And Breastfeeding: Postpartum Considerations

New moms, especially those with rheumatoid arthritis (RA), may experience a range of emotions and physical changes throughout the postpartum phase. While taking care of a newborn takes precedence, people with RA should also put their own health and well-being first during this period, especially as they deal with the difficulties of controlling their symptoms.

The possibility of RA flare-ups during the postpartum phase is one thing to take into account. Postpartum hormone fluctuations can exacerbate RA symptoms; some patients report flare-ups in the weeks or months after delivery. It's critical to watch out for indicators of elevated disease activity and, if necessary, seek emergency medical assistance.

Another thing to think about for RA patients who have recently given birth is breastfeeding. Although many RA drugs are thought to be safe to take while breastfeeding, it's important to talk to a healthcare professional about medication use to make sure that any drugs taken are safe for the unborn child. Medication changes can be required in certain situations to reduce exposure to the infant through breast milk.

Supportive actions can help new moms with RA deal with the difficulties of nursing while controlling their health.

Examples of these actions include contacting lactation support services and asking for help with childcare.

During this time, it's also critical to give self-care a high priority. This includes getting enough sleep, maintaining a good diet, and controlling stress.

During the postpartum phase, routine follow-up visits with healthcare experts are essential for monitoring RA symptoms, making any therapy adjustments, and addressing any potential issues.

Maintaining open lines of contact with medical professionals helps guarantee that any changes in a patient's condition are swiftly handled and that they get the assistance and care they require.

People with RA can confidently manage the postpartum time and concentrate on bonding with their new baby by prioritizing self-care, utilizing supportive resources, and maintaining communication with healthcare specialists. It is possible to properly manage RA symptoms and enjoy motherhood with the right assistance and care.

# CHAPTER SEVEN

## RHEUMATOID ARTHRITIS AND WORK

### Workplace Rights And Accommodations

Rheumatoid arthritis (RA) shouldn't prevent you from working. Knowing your rights and requesting the necessary modifications can have a big impact on how happy and productive you are at work. People with disabilities, including RA, are shielded against discrimination in the workplace by a number of regulations. Employers are required by the Rehabilitation Act of 1973 and the Americans with Disabilities Act (ADA) to make reasonable accommodations for eligible employees with disabilities, including those who have RA. Adjustments to occupational duties, ergonomic equipment, or changed work schedules are examples of reasonable accommodations.

## Techniques For Handling Stress And Fatigue Associated With Work

Managing fatigue and stress from work is essential for those with rheumatoid arthritis. Since stress can intensify RA symptoms, learning useful coping mechanisms is crucial. Stress levels can be controlled by setting priorities, engaging in relaxation exercises, and scheduling regular breaks in your work.

In addition, it's critical to counteract RA-related fatigue by getting enough sleep, exercising frequently, and maintaining a healthy work-life balance.

Open communication about your requirements and limitations with your employer can also assist reduce working stress and weariness.

## Interacting With Coworkers And Employers

Establishing a supportive work environment requires effective communication about your illness with employers and coworkers. You can encourage empathy and understanding by educating them about rheumatoid arthritis, its symptoms, and how it affects your capacity to work.

Communicate openly about your requirements and limitations, and talk about any accommodations that can improve your comfort and productivity at work. Promote candid communication and teamwork to identify solutions that satisfy all parties. Creating a network of coworkers who are understanding and considerate of your illness can also help reduce stress and foster a healthy work atmosphere.

# Benefits For Disability And Flexible Work Schedules

People with rheumatoid arthritis can greatly benefit from flexible employment arrangements.

Alternatives like job sharing, flexible scheduling, and telecommuting can assist in controlling pain and exhaustion as well as adapting to changing symptoms. Furthermore, if your illness keeps you from working a full-time job, knowing your rights to disability benefits like Supplemental Security Income (SSI) or Social Security Disability Insurance (SSDI) can help you financially. Investigate your options, speak with a disability advocate or lawyer, and make sure you understand the application procedure and get the benefits you are entitled to.

## Juggling Work-Related Obligations With Treatment And Self-Care

Effective management of rheumatoid arthritis requires juggling work obligations with self-care and medication. Make your health a priority by making frequent appointments with your physician, following your treatment regimen, and making time each day for self-care. This could involve physical therapy, exercise, rest, and stress-reduction methods. Be honest with your employer about the need for flexibility so that you can properly manage your health and attend medical appointments. Always keep in mind that your health comes first and that, in the end, caring for yourself helps you and your employer.

# CHAPTER EIGHT

## SCIENCE AND FUTURE POSSIBILITIES

### Current Research On Rheumatoid Arthritis Trends And Developments

The field of rheumatoid arthritis (RA) research is always changing in an effort to better understand and treat the condition.

The emphasis on personalized medicine, where therapies are customized for individual patients based on their distinct genetic makeup and illness features, is one noteworthy trend.

By choosing the most effective treatments and reducing side effects, this strategy seeks to maximize results.

The discovery of novel RA biomarkers is a crucial field of research. The identification of biomarkers, which are quantifiable signs of disease activity or progression, can result in early diagnosis and more specialized medical care. Scientists are investigating different blood tests, imaging methods, and molecular markers to enhance the diagnosis and tracking of RA.

The gut microbiome and its possible connection to RA have drawn more attention in recent years. Research indicates that abnormalities in gut flora could be a factor in autoimmune reactions and inflammation, which could result in the onset or aggravation of RA. Gaining insight into these relationships may lead to novel approaches to prevention and treatment.

Furthermore, new developments in imaging technologies have completely changed how RA is identified and tracked. Accurately assessing the activity and course of a disease is made easier for physicians by the comprehensive images of damaged joints that are provided by techniques like magnetic resonance imaging (MRI) and ultrasound.

## Potential Treatment Strategies In The Works

Exciting advancements in the treatment of RA are giving patients hope for better results and a higher quality of life. Using biological treatments, which target certain molecules involved in the inflammatory process, is one promising strategy. In several cases, biologics have demonstrated exceptional effectiveness in reducing joint degeneration and symptoms, even in patients who do not respond well to traditional treatments.

The use of small molecule inhibitors, which target intracellular signaling pathways implicated in the pathophysiology of RA, is another new therapeutic option. These medications are administered orally and may offer patients who are intolerant of biologics or do not respond to them an option.

Researchers are also looking into how regenerative medicine might be used to treat RA. For example, stem cell therapy shows promise in immune response modulation and joint tissue repair.

These novel techniques, however still in the early phases of development, have promising prospects for the treatment of RA in the future.

## Clinical Trials' Significance In Promoting Rheumatoid Arthritis Treatment

In order to assess the safety and effectiveness of novel RA medications and therapies, clinical studies are essential. The purpose of these meticulously planned and executed investigations is to collect empirical data that supports medical judgment.

Patients who take part in clinical trials can receive innovative therapies that aren't usually available to the general public quite yet.

Additionally, it advances scientific understanding by producing data that aids in the understanding of disease mechanisms and the testing of novel theories.

Strict ethical and legal guidelines are followed during clinical studies to guarantee patient safety and data integrity.

Prior to participation, informed agreement is sought from each participant, and they are continuously followed for the whole study.

Patients who take part in clinical trials not only help advance medical science but also get access to professional medical treatment and support from committed research teams.

## Campaigning And Collecting Money For Rheumatoid Arthritis Research

Raising awareness of RA and promoting financing for research and policy reforms are important tasks for advocacy organizations and patient advocacy groups.

These groups put in a lot of effort to inform the public, decision-makers, and medical professionals about the effects of RA on people and society at large.

By means of advocacy, patients with RA and their families may make their views heard, swaying policymakers to finance research at the top of the priority list and backing programs that enhance RA treatment and results.

Walks runs, and charity events are examples of fundraising activities that contribute to the much-needed funding for RA support services and research.

In addition to raising money, these gatherings help patients, carers, and supporters feel more connected to one another.

## Prospects For Enhanced Results And Life Quality For Patients With Rheumatoid Arthritis In The Future

Future prospects for RA care are very promising. It is anticipated that improvements in treatment options, research, and technology will improve the prognosis and quality of life for those who have the illness.

Approaches to personalized medicine will keep developing, enabling specialized care that takes into account the unique requirements and traits of every patient.

With its individualized approach, therapeutic efficacy could be maximized and side effects might be reduced.

In addition, continued study into disease mechanisms and biomarkers will enhance early identification and intervention, permitting prompt and focused treatments that can avert joint injury and impairment.

Medical device and assistive technology advancements will also improve the quality of life for RA patients by assisting them in managing their symptoms and preserving their independence.

All things considered, the future of RA is bright and moving forward thanks to ongoing cooperation between researchers, medical professionals, advocacy groups, and the RA community as a whole.

Together, we can work towards a time when RA is more fully recognized, properly treated, and eventually cured.

# CHAPTER NINE

## COMMONLY ASKED QUESTIONS OR FAQS

### How Does Rheumatoid Arthritis Develop?

The beginning of rheumatoid arthritis (RA) is a complicated illness that is influenced by several factors. It is thought to be caused by a confluence of immune system failure, environmental stimuli, and genetic predisposition, while the precise reason is yet unknown.

Due to the increased chance of acquiring RA in those with a family history of the condition, genetics play a major part in the disease. Some genetic markers have been linked to a higher risk of developing RA, including the HLA-DRB1 gene.

Environmental variables are also involved in the start of RA in persons who are genetically prone to the disease.

These elements could include exposure to certain contaminants, smoking, illnesses, and hormone fluctuations.

One of the main characteristics of RA is immune system dysfunction, which occurs when the body's immune cells attack healthy tissues—especially the synovium, which lines the joints—by mistake. This results in joint injury, persistent inflammation, and other systemic disease symptoms.

In an effort to better understand the underlying processes of RA, researchers are still delving into the complex interactions between immune dysfunction, genetics, and environment.

## Does Rheumatoid Arthritis Run In Families?

Yes, rheumatoid arthritis (RA) has a hereditary component. People who have a family history of RA are more likely to get the illness themselves. Having a family member with RA, however, does not ensure that you will have it as well.

Variations in the HLA-DRB1 gene, for example, are genetic markers linked to a higher risk of developing RA. However, the disease's start is not solely determined by genetics. The development of RA is also significantly influenced by immune system dysfunction and environmental variables.

Therefore, RA is not only inherited, even though genetics can predispose people to it. The disease's incidence and course are also influenced by other factors, including immune system malfunction and environmental stressors.

## Is There A Cure For Rheumatoid Arthritis?

There is yet no known treatment for the chronic inflammatory illness rheumatoid arthritis (RA). However, it is feasible to effectively manage the symptoms and slow down the disease's progression with an early diagnosis and suitable treatment.

Reducing inflammation, preserving joint function, easing pain, and enhancing the quality of life for RA patients are the main objectives of treatment. This frequently entails a mix of prescription drugs, dietary adjustments, and individually designed therapy.

Nonsteroidal anti-inflammatory drugs (NSAIDs), disease-modifying antirheumatic medications (DMARDs), biologic agents, and corticosteroids are among the medications frequently used to treat RA. These drugs aid in immune system suppression, inflammatory management, and joint preservation.

Apart from pharmaceutical interventions, lifestyle adjustments including consistent physical activity, physiotherapy, relaxation, and stress reduction can also aid in the treatment of RA symptoms and enhance general health. Sustaining a nutritious diet high in items that reduce inflammation and abstaining from smoking will help control RA even more.

Even though there isn't a cure for RA, research is still being done to improve outcomes for those who have this chronic illness by expanding our understanding of the illness and creating novel treatments.

## How Should I Handle Flare-Ups Of My Rheumatoid Arthritis?

Flare-ups of rheumatoid arthritis (RA), which are marked by increased joint pain, stiffness, edema, and exhaustion, can be difficult to control. To manage flare-ups when they happen and reduce their frequency and intensity, there are a few techniques that can be used.

Above all, it's critical to collaborate closely with your medical team to create a personalized treatment plan that suits your unique requirements and preferences. This could involve pain and inflammation-relieving drugs, lifestyle changes, and therapies to promote joint health and general well-being.

Rest and self-care must be given top priority during a flare-up. Taking care of yourself by listening to your body and not overdoing it can exacerbate pain and take longer to heal. Stretching and range-of-motion exercises are examples of gentle workouts that can assist enhance joint mobility and lessen stiffness without escalating inflammation.

During flare-ups, using cold or heat therapy on the afflicted joints can also help reduce pain and inflammation. Heat therapy helps relax muscles and increase blood flow to the joints, while cold packs assist numb the area and minimizing swelling.

Additionally, emotional stress can worsen the symptoms of RA. This can be prevented by engaging in stress-reduction practices including deep breathing, mindfulness, and meditation.

Having a strong support system of friends, family, and medical professionals by your side can also be a great way to get emotional support when flare-ups occur.

Despite the difficulties this chronic condition presents, you may enhance your overall quality of life and effectively manage RA flare-ups by putting these techniques into practice and collaborating closely with your healthcare team.

### If I Think I May Have Rheumatoid Arthritis, What Should I Do?

It's critical to get medical help right away if you think you may have rheumatoid arthritis (RA) or if you are exhibiting symptoms like weariness, stiffness, swelling, or joint pain. In order to properly manage RA and minimize joint deterioration and disability, early diagnosis and treatment are essential.

Making an appointment with your primary care physician or a rheumatologist—a medical professional who specializes in the diagnosis and treatment of rheumatic disorders, including arthritis—is the first step. In addition to reviewing your medical history and doing a physical examination, your doctor may conduct diagnostic tests, such as joint aspiration, imaging scans, or blood tests, to confirm the diagnosis during your visit.

Once you have been diagnosed with RA, your doctor will collaborate with you to create a personalized treatment plan that suits your requirements and preferences. This could involve lifestyle changes, physical therapy, and other therapies to maintain joint health and general well-being in addition to drugs to reduce pain and inflammation.

It's critical to educate yourself about RA and take an active role in your care in addition to receiving medical attention. Seek trustworthy information sources, pose inquiries, and be transparent with your medical team regarding your symptoms, worries, and desired course of therapy.

Living with RA can be difficult, but it is possible to manage the illness well and retain a high quality of life with early diagnosis, suitable therapy, and continued support. Never be afraid to ask for assistance and support when navigating your rheumatoid arthritis journey.

www.ingramcontent.com/pod-product-compliance
Lightning Source LLC
Chambersburg PA
CBHW071838210526
45479CB00001B/188